A.T.C. Pierson

Father of Minnesota Freemasonry

By Ray Hayward

Ray Hayward Enterprises, LLC

A.T.C. Pierson
Father of Minnesota Freemasonry

First Printing – 2018.

Photographs courtesy of Todd Jovonovich, Minnesota Masonic Historical Society, David Brewster, Wikipedia, and the author.

Published by: **Ray Hayward Enterprises, LLC**

Disclaimer: The author and publisher of this book are not responsible for any injury that may result from following the instructions contained herein. The reader should consult his or her physician for advice before attempting any such activities.

ISBN 978-0-692-03990-8

1 2 3 4 5 6 / 23 22 21 20 19 18

Table of Contents

Dedication

To the memory of ...

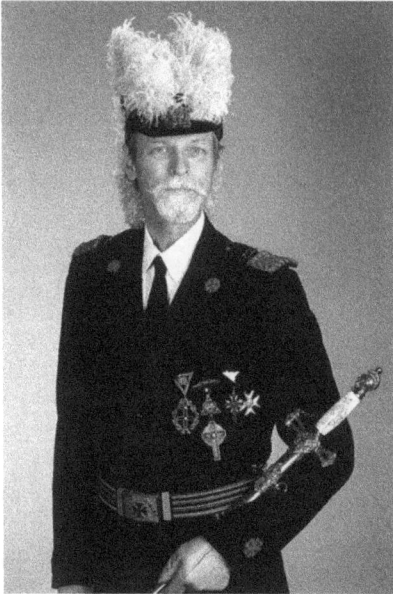

Sir Knight Charles W. Nelson
Right Eminent Past Grand
Commander of the
Grand Commandry of Knights
Templar of Minnesota
2000-2001

Acknowledgments

A very special thanks to:
Sir Knight Charles W. Nelson (R.I.P.), Past Grand Commander,
2000-2001
M.W.B. Judge David Sinclair Bouschor, Past Grand Master, 1988
W.B. Joseph Lang, Lodge Rosslyn-Sinclair 606
E.C. Todd Jovonovich P.H.P. Minnesota Chapter Number 1 RAM
E.C. Jack Roberts P.H.P. Minnesota Chapter Number 1 RAM
Companion Jack Morehouse 33rd Degree
Minnesota Masonic Museum and Historical Society
Sharon Nyberg, editor
Julie Cisler, design
David Brewster, photography

Foreword

by Dan Sherry

In the 150 years since A.T.C. Pierson became the Father of Minnesota Freemasonry, both the state of Minnesota and Freemasonry have seen good times and less-than-good times, even stressful times. Through it all, Freemasonry provided an unwavering fellowship of friends and caring that moderated those ebbs and flows of life. Even the Lodge itself became an enduring, physical safe haven, an oasis from outside stress.

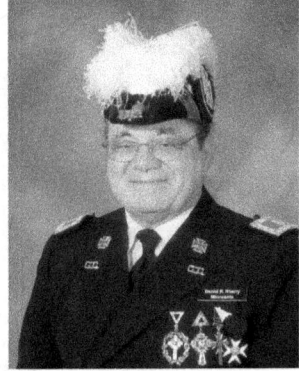

As the years have passed, other Masons have risen to replace A.T.C. Pierson and his generation. At the 125th anniversary of Minnesota Freemasonry, Charles Nelson honored the high principles of decades past. In turn, at the 150th anniversary, he passed the Freemasonry baton to outstanding new Masons, such as Ray Hayward. When the 175th anniversary arrives, perhaps sooner than we imagine, a new generation of Minnesota Freemasons will carry on the legacy of Freemasonry in the memory of A.T.C. Pierson, Charles Nelson and many others.

Minnesota Freemasonry will continue into the far distant future as a vibrant, long-term entity, where lasting friendships and leadership develop. Our future will always be passed by the symbolic baton from one Masonic generation to the next – and will continue to build upon and strengthen the cornerstone of A.T.C. Pierson.

Some of Dan Sherry's Knights Templar titles:
+ Grand Commander of the Grand Commandery of Knights Templar of Minnesota 2014-2015 and 2015-2016
+ North Central Dept. Commander 2018-2021

Foreword

by Timothy Warren Hogan

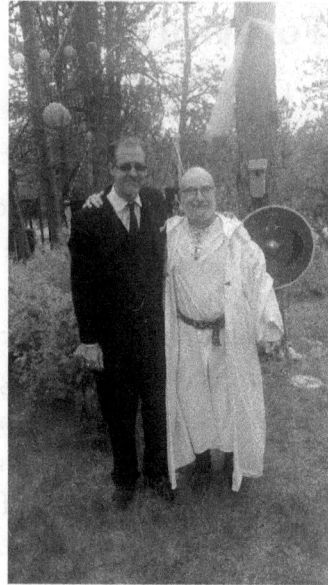

The United States of America has a great legacy due to the early foundation laid by Freemasons. At the beginning of this country, there were Masons who were endeavoring to not only build a new nation that was founded on Masonic ideals, but they were also working hard to bring elements of Freemasonry over from Europe. As Freemasonry started to grow in new soil, it required leaders who understood it's mysteries to become beacons of light, assisting in its growth and development, and framing its structure in new territories. The success of its mission in these territories demanded that the leaders could successfully communicate the tradition to new apprentices, and ultimately oversee new Masters as they propagated the degrees and the various Rites of the fraternity. Perhaps the greatest founding father and overseer of the work in the territory of Minnesota was A.T.C. Pierson. His understanding of the history and mysteries of Freemasonry, combined with his presence of leadership, allowed Freemasonry to take root in Minnesota, and to become established as a power nexus in the region. Beyond Minnesota Freemasonry, A.T.C. Pierson had an influence that extended throughout the United States, and attracted the attention of other notable figures of the time, including Albert Pike. A.T.C. Pierson's understanding of the Craft allowed him to publish works of value to other Freemasons, so that the tradition and mysteries of Freemasonry would be absorbed and preserved by those who were setting up the new American Masonic system.

The author of this book, Ray Hayward, has taken care to study as many materials as he could on A.T.C. Pierson, in order to provide a complete picture of the man who established so much for Minnesota Freemasonry. Ray Hayward's own study of the mysteries of Freemasonry has allowed him to have a full understanding of the motivation of A.T.C. Pierson, and has allowed him to appreciate the work that he was trying to perpetuate. In this way, Ray Hayward has been able to capture the essential aspects of this history in a way that few could.

I sincerely believe that this book will be of value to any Freemason who hopes to understand the motivation, history and tradition of early Freemasonry in Minnesota in particular, and in the United States in general. A.T.C. Pierson stood as a nexus point between old world Freemasonry trickling into the new United States of America, and the new systems of thought that were to take hold for the country. A.T.C. Pierson's influence extended beyond Minnesota and into other territories who shared common lineage. Ray Hayward has captured this moment in time in the following pages, and I invite you to be attentive to this light, as it speaks not only to Freemasonry's past, but to the essential qualities that can guide our collective Masonic future.

Most Fraternally In Light,
Timothy Warren Hogan
Grandmaster, Knights Templar O.T.S.I.

Foreword

By Judge David Sinclair Bouschor

A.T.C. Pierson, the cornerstone of Minnesota Masonry, was a giant in Freemasonry. Ray Hayward has presented him to us in a most pleasant and interesting manner. Pierson came to Minnesota to work for the Native Americans but soon discovered a great embezzlement by his superiors in the Indian Bureau. The manner in which he handled this immediately reflected his morality and honesty. He also, pursuant to a charter from the Grand Lodge of Ohio, came to found a Grand Lodge of Masonry in Minnesota. In 1853, he began to spread the Craft throughout the state. He granted many charters as Grand Master, but refused one where the applicants wanted to restrict membership to a nationality and language. His comment was that all Masonry is a common fraternity and "we should meet on one common Level, act by one common Plumb, and part upon one common Square." A.T.C. Pierson was a moral individual and devoted to the Craft. He also was instrumental in the beginnings of the York Rite and Scottish Rite. He was well respected by Albert Pike, founder of the Scottish Rite in America. In time, however, their egos kept them at arm's length throughout their lifetime. Of course Pierson and Pike had been loyal to opposite sides in the Civil War. This I am sure was a concern for both, but Masonry kept alive the friendship between them.

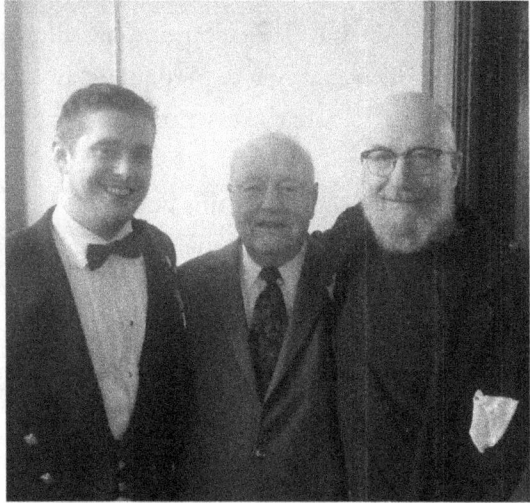

Ray Hayward has done a fine job of introducing our Grand Master Pierson of Minnesota, a fine citizen, and champion of our Native Americans. His philosophy was " Love one another, for that is the whole law."

Some of Judge Bouschor's Masonic Titles and achievements:

- Past Grand Master of the Grand Lodge of Masons of Minnesota, 1988
- Past Grand High Priest of the Grand Chapter of Royal Arch Masons of Minnesota, 1975
- Past Grand Illustrious Master of the Grand Council of Cryptic Masons of Minnesota, 1981
- Grand Piper of the Grand Commandery of Knights Templar of Minnesota 2011-2012
- 33rd A.A.S.R.
- Chief Adept (retired) of North Star College MSRICF
- Founder of Clan Sinclair USA

Introduction

I was introduced to A.T.C. Pierson by my mentor, brother, and friend, Charles W. Nelson. Charlie was not only an active Freemason and historian, he was also the chief historical architect for the state of Minnesota. He knew a lot about Pierson, who was one of his Masonic heroes, and he loved to tell facts, tidbits, and anecdotes about him. As a student of Charlie's and belonging to many of the same Masonic bodies and rites as both Charlie and A.T.C. Pierson, I also became fascinated with this "founding father" of Minnesota Freemasonry. Traveling around Minnesota I saw many historical documents and lodge charters with Pierson's signature.

Azariah Theodore Crane Pierson was born just after the founding of our country, which was based on Freemasonry. He was in a place of great influence and leadership during the Civil War. The nation's healing process began after the war with help from Freemasonry and Masons like A.T.C. Pierson.

This book started as a power-point lecture I gave with my friend and companion, Todd Jovonovich, at the 150th anniversary of the Grand Chapter of Royal Arch Masons of Minnesota, which was attended by past-General Grand High Priest Larry Gray. Most Excellent Grand Companion Gray encouraged me to expand my lecture into an article, or even a book. I also gave a version of this power-point and lecture at the 150th anniversary of the Grand Commandery of Knights Templar of Minnesota. The project of transforming this into a book sat for years, but now I am happy to say that I have finished it, at least my small part of the telling.

This is the story of not only a well-read and accomplished Freemason but also an extraordinary American citizen — one who lived in interesting times and who wrestled with many obstacles, both personally and collectively as an American and as a Freemason. I don't intend this book to be a "tell-all" biography but a glimpse and insight into an extraordinary life. It is my intention, however, to introduce one of my personal heroes and examples of the integrity known as being a member of "the Craft."

> "The true Mason is an ardent seeker after knowledge, and he knows that books are vessels which come down to us full freighted with the intellectual relics of the past."
> - A.T.C. Pierson

1
Early Life

"Masonry is a progressive science; all its mysterious light, all its sublime truths are not at once developed; it is only by gradual steps that its beauties are unfolded to the wondering mind of the aspirant."
- A.T.C. Pierson

Azariah Theodore Crane Pierson was born Aug. 29, 1817, in Speedwell, near Morris Plains, New Jersey. The son of Joseph B. Pierson, he was a descendant of Abraham Pierson and Jasper Crane, two families from a group of Puritans who founded Montclair, New Jersey, in 1666. Pierson's family moved to Cincinnati, Ohio, when he was 4, then back to New Jersey after a year. They finally settled in New York a few years later. Pierson was educated in New York.

At age 18, he married 16-year-old Eleanor C. Berrien, daughter of James Berrien of Herlgate, Long Island. It was a marriage that would last 54 years. They had three daughters. In 1837, at age 20, he graduated from the Barclay Street Medical College in New York. He made his living as a traveling druggist-supply salesman.

Pierson came to St. Paul, Minnesota, in 1851 to take a job as a confidential clerk for the superintendent of the Indian Department, working with the Winnebago, Chippewa, and Sioux tribes. He held that position until the controversies — land grabs, broken treaties, subjugation — that lead to the Indian outbreak of 1862.

As superintendent of schools on several reservations, Pierson uncovered that his superiors were embezzling money from Native American schoolchildren. The theft of about $5,000 resulted in the resignation or dismissal of those officials. Known as the Chippewa Disturbance, this fraud led to many uprisings in Minnesota. Pierson left the Indian Bureau and was appointed chief draftsman for the Surveyor General of the city of St. Paul.

> "A month later Galbraith (corrupt Indian Bureau agent) was fearful that the superintendent of schools on the reservation, ATC Pierson, had discovered that the agency had lost not less than $5,000 between August 1860 and January 1862."
> *Chief Hole-in-the-Day and the 1862 Chippewa Disturbance, a reappraisal by Mark Diedrich*

Here is a description of Pierson from a book, *Pen Pictures of St. Paul and Biographical Sketches of Old Settlers 1859* ,about the early settlers and founders of the State of Minnesota:

> "Who is that man with the long hair and a slouch hat, and a swaggering motion, and who moves his head rapidly from one side to another, and thrusts his hands deep down into the pockets of his pants? That is A.T.C. Pierson, the great Mason, who has climbed the Morgan ladder to the top round and is looking about to see if he can't grapple with the stars and steal into the otherworld and establish a higher order of Masonry there. He is as young in feeling and in action as a boy of sixteen, and yet he makes a splendid picture of a grand old patriarch as he really is, just stepping upon the last step which leads to three score and ten. His flowing locks, his elastic step, his rapid movements, his boyish yet venerable appearance, all make him a paradoxism [sic]– a sort of contradiction, and yet as a whole he is com-

plete and individualized into an exception to a general rule; in a word, he is a character! There are very few, if any, men in the country better posted on Masonry than Pierson, as he has made it a life study and has written several books on the subject, and if Masonry is as grand and sublime as its advocates claim it is, Mr. Pierson ought to be good enough to go to heaven on a sunbeam: if he isn't, he's to blame, not Masonry. Mr. Pierson is a fine-looking man and his portrait presents a striking appearance. He is social in his nature, and outwardly, is all one needs to ask for when dealing 'on the square.'"

2
Masonic Life

A.T.C. Pierson "was a profound student of Masonry and very few have grasped the spirit and gained the knowledge he possessed of its laws and traditions in so short a time."
- Edward Johnstone

Pierson pursued Freemasonry after hearing a public speech by General Lafayette on the subject in 1824. Pierson was raised as a Master Mason in Painted Post Lodge No. 117, New York in 1851. He entered Minnesota Freemasonry life on Feb. 7, 1853, acting as proxy for the Grand Master of Ohio to install and duly constitute the first lodges. He was involved in bringing all the Grand Bodies of Freemasonry to Minnesota.

> "Freemasonry is an order whose leading star is philanthropy, and whose principles inculcate an unceasing devotion to the cause of virtue and morality."
> *-Brother Gilbert du Motier, Marquis de Lafayette*

Pierson was a charter member of Ancient Landmark No. 5 and served as Junior Warden, the highest office he held in that lodge. Indeed, for Pierson to act in the capacity of a past master, he relied on his "virtual past master" from Royal Arch Masonry.

He was elected the third Grand Master, serving nine years in that office. Pierson is the only Grand Master who wasn't a Master of a lodge. Forty-one lodges were chartered during his time as Grand

Master, the most any Grand Master opened. He also closed more lodges because whole memberships died in the Civil War.

Pierson served the Grand Lodge of Minnesota during a period of great stress and strife. New lodges were chartered every year, and he visited each of them during a period when transportation was limited to horseback or boat. The first train service didn't start until 1862, when 10 miles of track were opened between St. Paul and St. Anthony. Communication was limited to mail service and the telegraph. The economic depression of 1859 and the coming Civil War also complicated attempts to firmly establish Masonry in Minnesota. Many blue lodges experienced difficulties during the Civil War as members left for military service. Scottish Rite activity was virtually nonexistent during the war years.

> "Not a company has gone from this State but that some of our Lodges were represented in it (the Civil War); not a regiment but that at least half of its officers were members of our Order; not a Lodge in the State but that some of its officers have answered their country's call. In some of the our Lodges, one year since, all the officers had gone; in others, a portion of the officers and members, and in one Lodge but three members were left."
>
> -A.T.C.Pierson, Grand Master, Annual Communication, October 1863

Although Pierson granted many charters, there was one that he declined. Many German immigrants moved to Minnesota during its early years. When Pierson received the petition to establish a German-only speaking lodge, he denied it, by saying:

> "No act should be done or recognized which will affect or tend to produce a cast of country or character among those who, as one common Fraternity, should meet

18

upon one common level, act by one common plumb, and part upon one common square."

In his day, Pierson met the challenges that immigration and language posed to the fledgling state, and sought unity and harmony above all.

He also laid the foundation for the recognition of African-American Freemasonry, known as Prince Hall Masonry, by weighing in and defending the Prince Hall Masons as "regular" as opposed to "irregular." It has been debated for years whether African-American Masons were "irregular," or merely "clandestine." Irregular implied not balanced, contrary, or not properly arranged, as opposed to clandestine which meant hidden or secret. Pierson found their rites, rituals, and Craft to be correct, sound, and legitimate.

Communication between Pierson and various Grand Lodges and Bodies reveal his wealth of knowledge, good manners, humor, and personality. It also shows the respect he gave, and was shown. The following letter to the Grand Lodge of Louisiana exemplifies his skill as a communicator.

TIDINGS FROM MINNESOTA.
St. Paul, Jan.15th, 1856.

Bro. Moore:—

This is a large country up here, and we are a fast people, and growing some, although pretty much froze out since Christmas. Cold? I guess you would have thought so, had you been here; lucky for us the thermometer was no longer on the lower end, — mercury "squatted" (thousands do here) away down in the bottom; hid away; got scared; rolled up into a little ball and staid [sic] there. But cold as it was, the delegates to our Grand Lodge were prompt. Roll call found each Lodge (six) represented; some from a two days ride distant. (Therm. 30° below zero.) Is there not an exemplification of the love of Masonry way up north here among the Indians, that proves we have worthy Masons among us? We do not pay our delegates!

We were in session four days. The utmost harmony and entire unanimity characterized all our proceedings. Three new Charters were granted, and a new Constitution adopted.

Grand Master Sherburne's address is a very able Masonic document, and will excite considerable attention, particularly that portion which relates to Confederation. He recommends a General Representative body, with appellate jurisdiction only, to be composed of one Representative from each Grand Lodge; his actual expenses to be paid by his Grand Lodge; said body to meet once in two, three, or four years, only when necessity should require — no new titles.

I will send you the proceedings as soon as they are published.

The Order is in a very flourishing condition in this Territory. Two applications are now before me for dispensations for new Lodges. Two years since in those localities, the only residents were the Red Men of the Prairie; and now, although the land has not yet been surveyed by government, from 80 to 75 miles west of the Mississippi River, there are flourishing towns, in one, 19 Masons, in another 11 Masons.

A brother traveling through the country south of the Minnesota River to the Iowa line, from the Mississippi River west, will find many a Bro, Comp, and Sir

KT. I have been surprised, time and again, in traveling over our broad prairies, or through the woods, to come upon a small log house, 10,15, 20 miles from any other house, to find the occupant a Bro, Comp, or Sir KT. They come to us from every state in the Union, from Canada, from Europe, from everywhere. About one half of our Territorial Legislative are of the same stamp.

Bro. Moore come up and see us: go over the prairies with me; view our beautiful lakes, forests and broad streams. Visit the log-huts, shantys and &c. You will find the rough dressed backwoodsman, one who has visited the inner courts; who remembers well, what he saw, heard, and felt; that other one has passed the circle of perfection, and is very circumspect; secrecy and silence he regards as virtues, but his eyes glisten at the sight of a square, and will talk of the Book of the Law, or Ark of the Covenant; but speak to him of Constantine's vision, and he will take you to his heart. His cabin, his team, anything you require in his power to grant, is done for the word. Such, Bro, Moore, are a large portion of Minnesota Masons. Warm hearts, open hands, and faithful breasts. Come and see.

Don't understand me as claiming any merit, for warms hearts, &c, 'tis legitimate. Masons of necessity must be so, if they are Masons. I have traveled extensively, and never yet found an asylum closed to the stranger, and such as was had or required, was freely given.

Fraternally Yours, &c, &c,
A.T.C. Pierson

Pierson was elected Grand Secretary for one term in 1856, and then served as Grand Secretary from 1876 until his death in 1889.

He organized and taught the Masonic ritual throughout the state and hand copied ciphers for all the Masonic bodies. He traveled extensively to instruct lodges in the work and general running of the craft. He would be gone for days, traveling by riverboat, wagon, or horseback to reach his destination. Pierson unified the Preston-Webb Masonic Ritual work and, in order to identify it, his Masonic students referred to it as the "Pierson Work."

> "We think that those who hold fast to the oldest forms
> of ritual are entitled to the most credit, and not the
> ones who have shown the most inventive genius and
> have the greatest 'improvements'. We are constitution-
> ally opposed to changes and experiments in Masonic
> Work. We generally find the improvements only to be
> changes, and that for the worse."
> -A.T.C. Pierson

Pierson amassed a huge library of Masonic, esoteric, and historical titles. His numerous reports and correspondences to various Grand Bodies reveal his broad and well-read Masonic education. He also authored two books on Freemasonry:

Traditions of Freemasonry and its Coincidences with the
Ancient Mysteries

The Traditions, Origin, and Early History of Freemasonry
(with Godfrey W. Steinbrenner).

He is featured in the Masonic Sketch Book and Gleanings from the Harvest Field of Masonic Literature by Edwin Du Laurans. In 1889 George R. Metcalf notified Albert Pike that he was sending the books of A.T.C. Pierson to Pike.

Here is how Pierson describes the frontispiece of his book, *Traditions of Freemasonry and its Coincidences with the Ancient Mysteries* (see page 41):

"Perhaps a few words of explanation about the frontispiece would not be amiss. The design represents the front of the Mystic Temple. The entrance is gained by seven steps; the entablature is supported by two columns; by each column stands the Guardian, the one a Mason, the other an Egyptian Priest who is lifting the veil that conceals the great mystery, which is symbolized by the Ineffable Name within a delta surrounded by a raise. Within are three groups of figures. In the center group, three people are standing around a prostrate figure and holding Masonic emblems – a rule, a square and a Hiram. The group on the right represents the perfidy of Typhon, enclosing his brother Osiris in a box. On the left side are two figures representing Cain and Abel – the archetype of the legend and all the mysteries. In front of the entablature is the Mystic cherubim described by Ezekiel, the winged bull of Nimroud, which is also depicted in the monuments of Egypt. An ancient altar on the opposite corner, and the symbol of Fraternity and the center figures of Hope and Charity at the base of the columns, with Faith in the center of the entablature; and the emblems — corn, wine, and oil — on each side; at the foot of the steps of grave, beside it lie certain tools, at the head of the grave, the emblem of Immortality."

3

York Rite

"What is it that induced you, my brethren, to leave your families, travel hundreds of miles? What inducement for this sacrifice of time, money, and ease? What, but the love of your fellow men – your desire to counsel together to advance the interests of Freemasonry."

- A.T.C. Pierson

Pierson assisted at the organization of the Grand Chapter of Royal Arch Masons of Minnesota in 1859 and was its first Grand High Priest. He was Secretary of the Grand Chapter from 1860 to 1864, inclusive, and 10 years later, accepted the office again and held it for the next 14 years until his death. He was General Grand King of the General Grand Chapter of Royal Arch Masons of the United States for three years. A Royal Arch Masonic Chapter was founded and named after him in Crookston, Minnesota: Pierson Chapter # 41 RAM

A.T.C. Pierson was exalted a Royal Arch Mason (RAM) at Elmira Chapter No. 42, Elmira, N.Y. He founded Minnesota Chapter No. 1 RAM along with many of the early leaders in Minnesota history, and was elected its first High Priest. It is interesting to note that the Chapter Penny for Minnesota Chapter No. 1 RAM and the State Seal of Minnesota are identical. That is because the founders of the chapter and of the state were the same men. It is the only Masonic Chapter Penny in the world that bears a state seal. Pierson's own personal mark reveals his reverence in connection with Native Americans and his sincere desire for peace.

General Grand High Priest Albert Mackey granted Minnesota a charter for its Grand Chapter in 1859. A.T.C. Pierson was elected the first Grand High Priest of Minnesota.

In 1866, Pierson was elected the first Excellent President of the Minnesota Order of High Priesthood. He was also appointed as Grand Lecturer "to disseminate the [ritual] work adopted by the Grand Chapter of Royal Arch Masons of Minnesota."

He holds the distinction of being the first High Priest, first Grand High Priest, and first Excellent President in Minnesota. His address to the first Grand Convocation of the Grand Chapter of Royal Arch Masons of Minnesota ends with this quote:" Love one another, for that is the whole law."

> "The first Grand High Priest of Minnesota was A.T.C. Pierson, a Freemason of conspicuous ability, who achieved a national reputation in every grade of Free-masonry in the American Rite."
>
> - Henry Leonard Stillson

Yet, with all of Pierson's involvement and accomplishments in the York Rite, he is not listed as a member of the Cryptic Council. This could be due to some controversy over the degrees and the development of that body. It seems that the Royal and Select Master degrees were considered side degrees by the Scottish Rite in America. At some point, Albert Pike no longer held them under his jurisdiction. But in Minnesota, Pierson was still awarding those degrees under the authority of Scottish Rite. This seems to be a bone of contention between two giants in the Masonic world. We have an excerpt from one of the meetings where Albert Pike states his complaints about Pierson and what was to become the Cryptic Council degrees;

> "Very Dear Brethren: Having heard that Ill.' Bro.' A. T. C. Pierson, 33d, late Grand Prior of the Supreme Council, still confers the degrees of the said Rite, and those of Royal and Select Master, in the State of Min-

nesota, and receives the fees therefore, we do deem it necessary to make it known unto you that the said Ill.' Bro.' resigned his membership in our Supreme Council at the session held in Baltimore on the 2nd day of May last, and has since then been only an Honorary Member thereof; and that he has since then had, and now has, no power or authority whatever to confer degrees or create bodies, of said Rite, or to confer the degrees of Royal and Select Master, or to receive moneys for degrees, in the State of Minnesota or elsewhere; and that all his acts so done since said session of our Supreme Council are null and void, and without the knowledge or authority of our Supreme Council.

And we do further give you to know that at the same session our Supreme Council formally relinquished all control over the degrees of Royal and Select Master, and that since that time none of our Inspectors General could lawfully invest any one with those degrees. And as the said Ill.' Bro.' has never reported to us any of his doings as Inspector General in Minnesota or elsewhere. We do advise those who have received from him any of the degrees of the said Rite to furnish us with the evidence thereof, that they may, if invested with them before our last session, receive the proper credentials whereby to prove lawful possession of the said degrees."

- Albert Pike

A.T.C. Pierson led the move to form the first Commandery of Knights Templar in Minnesota, Damascus Commandery No. 1. He was elected commander and served for nine years. Pierson served as recorder for Damascus Commandery No. 1 until he died. Elected Grand Recorder for the Grand Commandery of Minnesota in 1877, he also served in that position until his death in 1889.

Pierson was Grand Captain General of the Grand Encampment of Knights Templar of the United States of America from 1862-1868. He also is listed in the Grand Encampment records for the 15th Triennial as XV 1862 Azariah T.C. Pierson, St. Paul, Minnesota.

> "Companion Pierson, Grand Secretary, presented the report on foreign correspondents, which, like all of his, shows the 'Mark' in a true craftsman. Our proceedings for the 1886 (annual conclave) receive more than average attention, and he [Pierson] concurs with us in some of our reviews, which is gratifying to us indeed. There is no one whose opinion, Masonically, we trust in more than his."
>
> - *Grand High Priest W.F. Dickinson, 1887*

4
Scottish Rite

"A.T.C. Pierson made himself known to me as a Mason, at the village of St. Paul, in the territory of Minnesota, where he then resided. A mutual liking and occasional meetings followed, and our acquaintance ripened a few years afterwards into a friendship that lasted until he died. Ours was an acquaintance that was often strained, but never broken."
- Albert Pike

When Minnesota was transitioning from a territory into statehood in the 1850s, Pierson was busy bringing in as many Masonic bodies as he could. At the time, the country was split over such political differences as states rights and slavery. Many Minnesotans favored having the northern jurisdiction of the ancient and accepted Scottish Rite as the governing body for the Scottish Rite in Minnesota, as had their neighbor, Wisconsin. Pierson argued that politics and the location of the Sovereign Grand Commander, who was in the South, had nothing to do with Freemasonry. Pierson felt that Albert Pike and his southern jurisdiction had better rituals and education, and assisted Pike in spreading the Southern Jurisdiction of Scottish Rite to Nebraska, Kansas, and Nevada.

"It will be absolutely necessary that some of us should take in hand the dissemination of the Rite, as soon as the Rituals are ready. If we would affect anything, we must be willing to give our time and labour to the Order. I hope to induce our Ill.' Bro' Pierson to undertake the propagation of the Rite in Minnesota, Nebraska, Kansas and Nevada."

- *Albert Pike*

Pierson also felt an affinity for Pike. They seemed to be cut from the same cloth not only in appearance but also in their scholarly pursuits and love for the craft. Albert Pike came to Minnesota to personally communicate the fourth through the 32nd Degrees of the Scottish Rite to A.T.C. Pierson, who then received his 33rd Degree in Chicago in 1859.

Pierson was the first Sovereign Grand Inspector General for Minnesota. He served as Lieutenant Grand Commander in 1865, with Pike serving as Sovereign Grand Commander, and the famous Masonic scholar Albert Mackey as Secretary General, holding that third-highest office for life. Pierson was also Grand Prior of the Supreme Council.

A.T.C. Pierson, 33rd Degree, and Benjamin B. French, 33rd Degree, both active members of the Supreme Council, S.J., communicated the 4th to 32nd degrees to Andrew Johnson, the 17th U.S. President. Benjamin B. French was Grand Master of Masons in Washington, a 33rd degree Scottish Rite Mason, Grand Master of the Grand Encampment of Knights Templar, clerk of the House of Representatives, and the Commissioner of Public Buildings (including the United States Capitol and all federal Buildings). Johnson was the first president to become a Scottish Rite Mason, and he received those degrees in the White House on June 20, 1867. It should be noted that it was President Johnson who pardoned General Albert Pike for his support of the Confederacy. Pierson collected 67 signatures from prominent Masons for the petition to pardon Pike, and personally delivered it to Johnson.

The following is from the book: *Letters of President Johnson [Washington, D.C.]* June 18th. 1867

My Dear Sir & Brother.

The Supreme Council of the Ancient & Accepted Scottish Rite of the Southern Jurisdiction of the U.S. have been long desirous of placing you on their roll of Chiefs of that Order. They cannot do it however unless you are a 32d of that Rite, and only then by election at a regular meeting of that Body.

It is our wish now that you should possess the 32d Degree before going to Boston, and Brother A.T.C. Pierson being now in this City, if it should be your pleasure to become a 32d, we can make you one in a short time, occupying not over one hour.

It can be done privately too, that no one need know when you received the degrees, but it will only be known, after it, that you are a 32d.

Brother Pierson has been with me this morning, and proposes to call on you tomorrow morning to ascertain your wishes as to this matter, and I write this note that you may give the matter some thought before we see you.

B.B. French 33d
Sov. G. ‹Ins.› ‘Gen.› for the Dist. Of Columbia

Pierson's and Pike's relationship gradually became strained. As Pike had said, theirs was "an acquaintance that was often strained, but never broken." There were a few bones of contention, but I suspect that at the heart of their tension is that they were too much alike, and their personalities just couldn't bear a rival or competitor of the same ilk.

One of the issues that Pike reprimanded Pierson for was chartering a lodge in 1867 that he named after himself, the Pierson Lodge of Perfection. It seems you were only supposed to use the names of people who were deceased!

Another issue was that Pierson distributed illegal handwritten copies of ciphers, for which he received a public reprimand at the Southern Jurisdiction's annual meeting. Also Pierson may have thwarted Pike's move to have Minnesota's first three degrees be from Scottish Rite, as opposed to the established York Rite.

But the major reason that Pierson fell out of favor with Pike was because Pierson felt that the Scottish Rite was a graduate level of Masonic ritual and education. He also felt that it built upon the previous rites and rituals and opened men's minds to form their own opinions from their experiences.

With the growing popularity of the Scottish Rite in Minnesota, Pierson was against having any more than one candidate at a time go through the ranks and rituals while Pike introduced the idea of a "class" initiation, where one candidate went through the full ritual of initiation while all the others experienced it vicariously, sitting on the sidelines. Pierson felt every man should have his own experience of the degrees. This was echoed in the words of M.E.C. Thomas Montgomery, Grand High Priest of Minnesota in 1880;

"I insist that there is a wealth of meaning in all our ceremonies, that there symbolic teachings are simply sublime, and that no candidate should be deprived of the full benefit of that to which he is justly entitled."

In addition, Pierson was conferring degrees and not reporting them as accurately as required. He was not alone. Some of his brother Sovereign Grand Inspector Generals were also delinquent in their reporting. At this time, Pierson was traveling all over the Upper Midwest, spreading the light of Freemasonry. In his very own St. Paul Valley of Scottish Rite, some members wrote to Pike accusing Pierson of planning to found a new jurisdiction and make himself the Grand Commander. Many members of the St. Paul Valley defended Pierson and protested that he was being unfairly accused.

Pierson resigned from the Scottish Rite on April 13, 1870, at the Supreme Council session in Baltimore. His name was removed from the roster of the 33rd Degree and he lost his membership in the rite. Pierson then focused the remaining years of his Masonic career on the York Rite. He still remained active in the St. Paul Valley and quietly continued his work in the Scottish Rite there. The love and respect the St. Paul Valley held for Pierson is visible today for he is still listed on the roles as an honorary 33rd Degree member.

5
Legacy

"Pierson was a wise counselor, while learned in the Constitution, laws, and usages of masonry. He was also a profound student of the 'ancient work,' and taught it to the lodges."
- Edward Johnstone

After retiring as Grand Master, Pierson was referred to as "Father Pierson." He died on Nov. 26, 1889, at age 72, after a brief illness. He was buried with every Masonic honor and ceremony at Oakland Cemetery in St. Paul. The Saint Paul Globe reported his death saying:

The Saint Paul Globe

Nov. 29th

The funeral of A. T. C. Pierson.

> "grand recorder of the grand commandery of Knights Templar, whose death occurred on Tuesday last, will be held from the People's 'church' at 2 o'clock today. Special rates have been given on all roads running into the city, am —. a large contingent of Masons will be present from all parts of the country."

After his death, Eleanor "Mother" Pierson donated his vast library to the Grand Lodge, which revealed the depth and breadth of this extremely well-read Freemason. In her lifetime, Eleanor supported her husband's ritual work by sewing costumes and making paraphernalia for many Masonic organizations. She was awarded a jewel by the Masonic Veterans Association in loving remembrance of her service to the men in the craft. After her death in 1909, the Grand Lodge honored her and the "Father of Minnesota Masonry" with a monument.

From a newspaper clipping of Mother Pierson's death

MRS. E. C. PIERSON DEAD.
Widow of Prominent Minnesota Mason Passes Away.
St. Paul, Sept. 28.
— Mrs. Eleanor Pierson, aged eighty-six, widow of the late A. T. C. Pierson, who was prominent in the Masonic history of Minnesota, died Sunday at her home, 270 Dayton Avenue.

> "His name has been familiar throughout the American Masonic world for many years, and he has been connected in a prominent way with all the Masonic organizations of this state from the beginning."
>
> *- Grand Master J.A. Kiester in his address to the Grand Lodge of Minnesota in 1890, reporting on the death of Brother A.T.C. Pierson.*

Afterword

"Masonry adapts itself to circumstances, thus we have a different arrangement from that of our fathers, and yet the landmarks are the same."
- A.T.C. Pierson

Azariah Theodore Crane Peirson was a man who was in love with the Craft of Freemasonry. Ritual, history, the quest for light, and brotherly love were near and dear to his heart. He also wrestled with many of the difficult issues of his day: racism, divisiveness, oppression, deception, immigration, greed, injustice, despair, and the age-old meaning of life. He balanced and managed these issues with acceptance, truth, hope, justice, equality, integrity, equality, education, and self-realization — the tools he acquired from Freemasonry, personal study, and his life. We are still struggling with many of those issues today.

Pierson's life shows us how to rise above base thought and selfishness to not only survive, but also to thrive. I have seen Freemasonry go through many changes, some for the better, and some not so good. And not just Freemasonry, but every aspect of life. These rapid changes are almost mind boggling. And then out of the light of history, we see that change is nothing new. The only thing that doesn't change IS change!

I believe Freemasonry has the keys to a well-lived and prosperous life. I have experienced it in my life. I have seen the benefit in many others' lives. And I have studied it in A.T.C. Person's life. I have hope that the message of Freemasonry will live on.

> Where can those of good hearts and strong minds go for self-knowledge? To increase the light they have found within? To be of service to themselves and others? Go to lodge. A.T.C. Pierson set the cornerstone for us all.
>
> - Ray Hayward

Photo Gallery

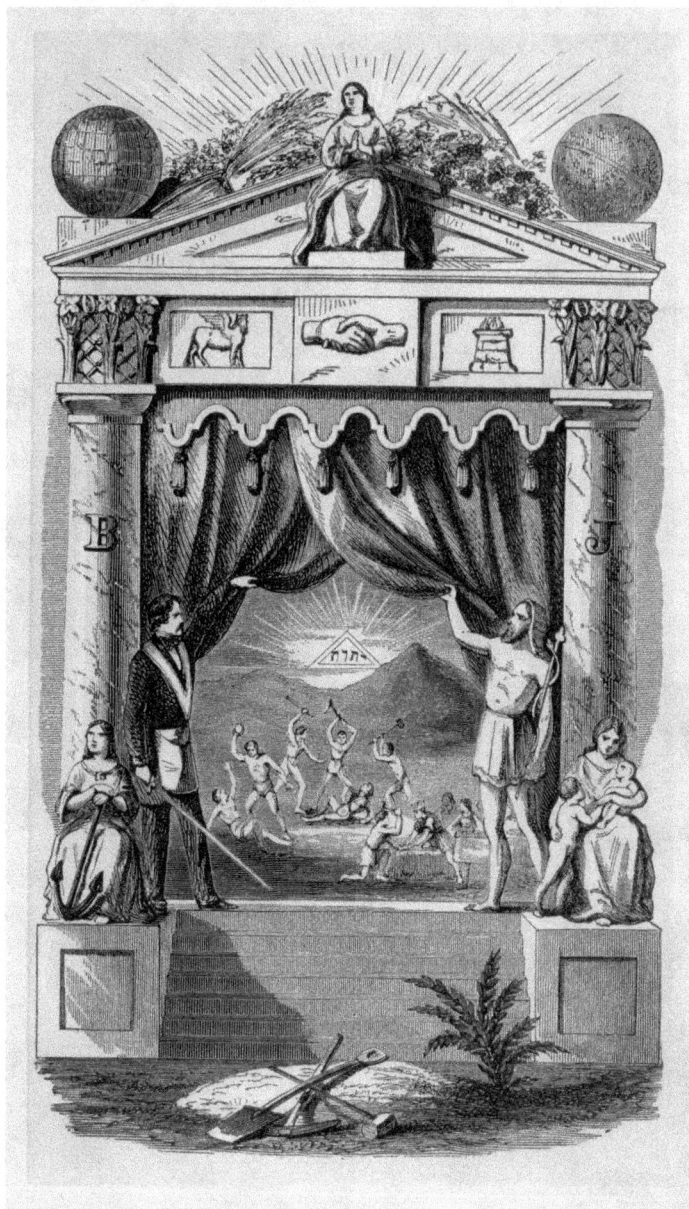

The Frontispiece of Pierson's book, Traditions of Freemasonry.

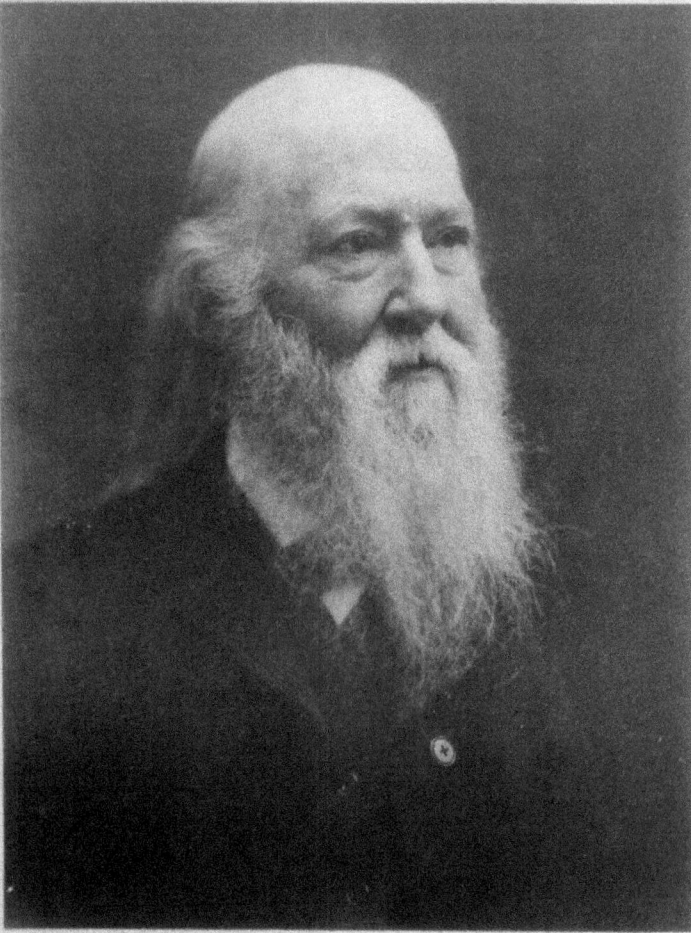

AZARIAH THEODORE CRANE PIERSON
ANCIENT LANDMARK LODGE NO. 5, ST. PAUL
GRAND MASTER, JAN. 1856 TO OCT. 1864
BORN 1817   DIED 1889

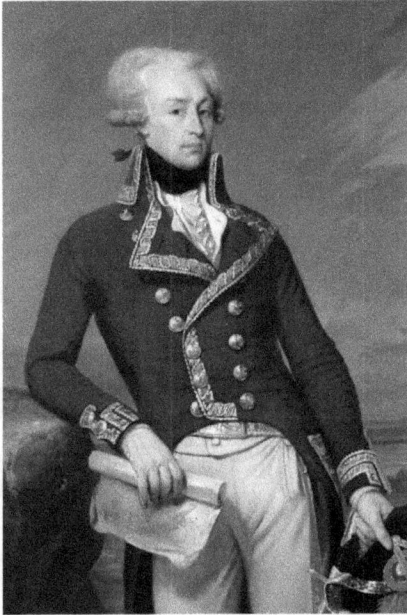

General Lafayette.

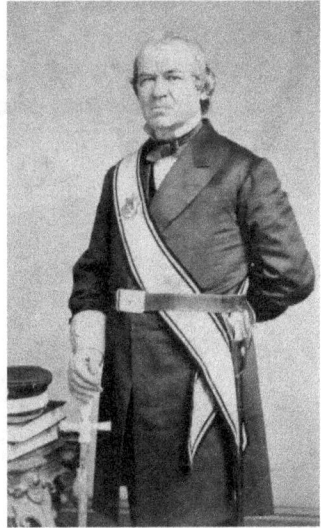

President Andrew Johnson, in
Knights Templar uniform.

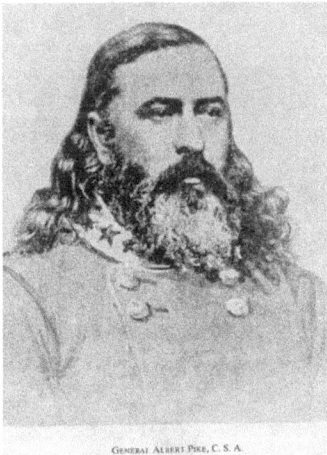

GENERAL ALBERT PIKE, C. S. A.

Albert Pike in Confederate uniform.

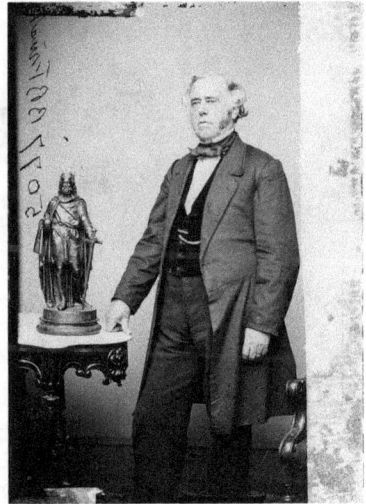

Benjamin B. French.

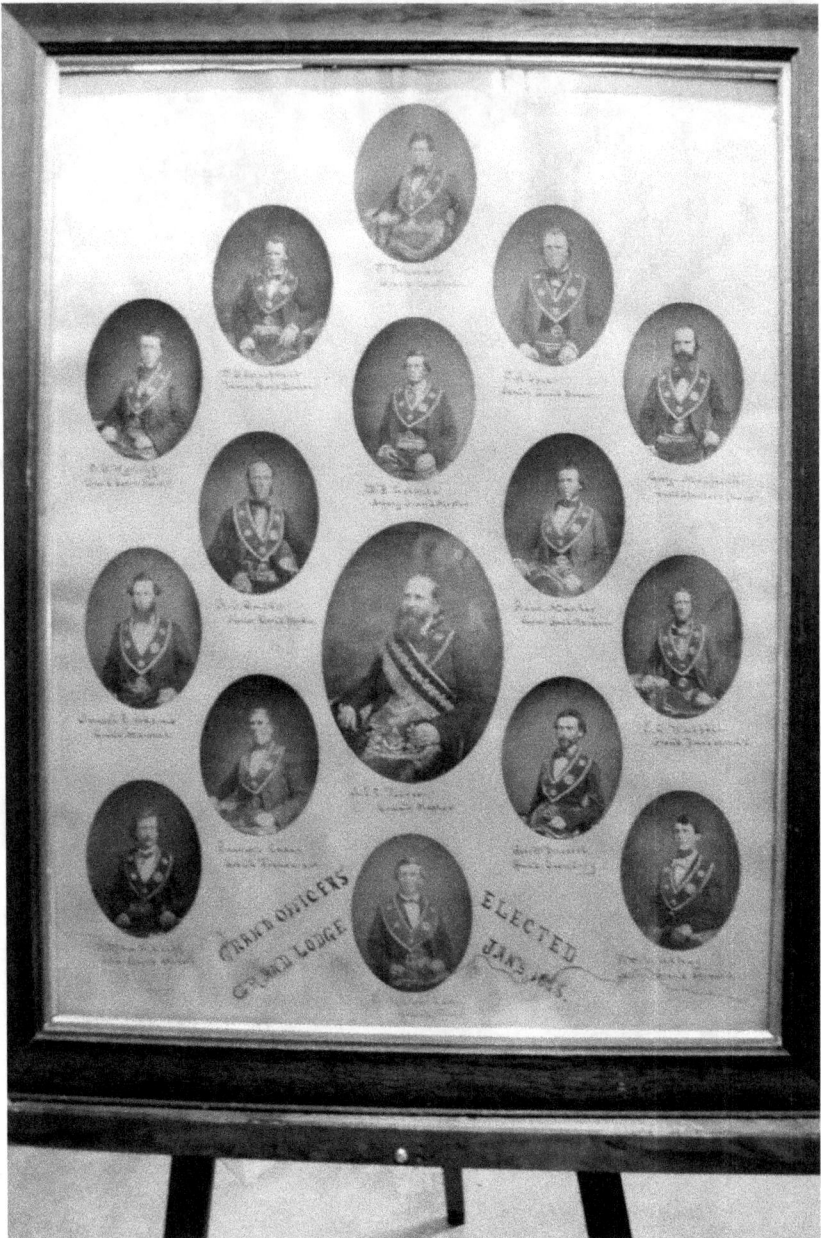

Grand Lodge officers of Minnesota with A.T.C. Pierson as Grandmaster in the middle.

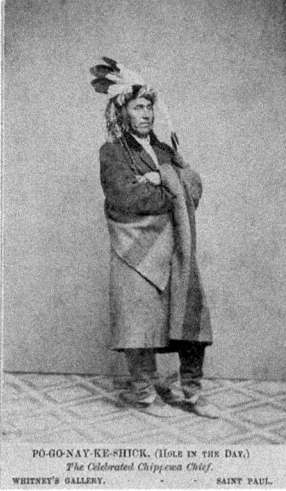

Chief Hole-in-the-Day.

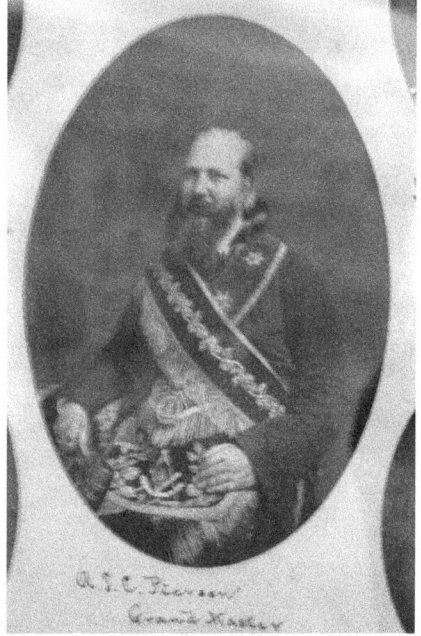

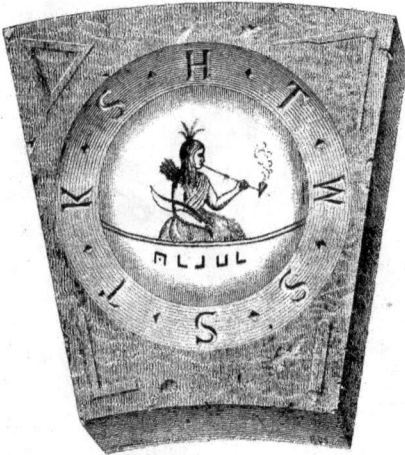

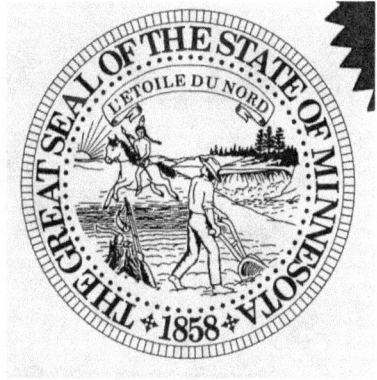

Pierson's "Mark" showing RAM cipher and Native American smoking peace pipe.

EARLY SETTLERS

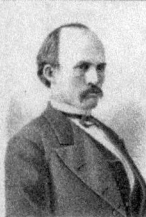

HENRY S. BASSETT.
Preston.

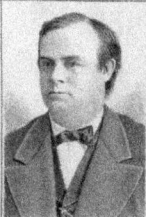

THOMAS SIMPSON.
Winona.

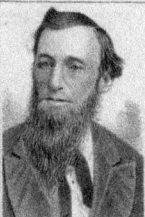

A. J. STEVENS.
Rushford.

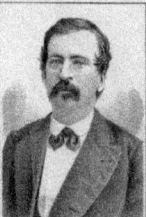

A. W. WHITE.
Albert Lea.

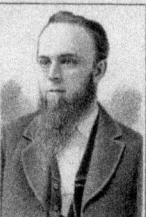

H. D. BROWN.
Albert Lea.

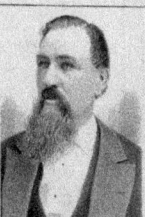

W. H. DILL.
Winona.

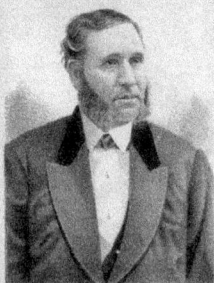

W. C. MORRISON Esq.
St. Paul.

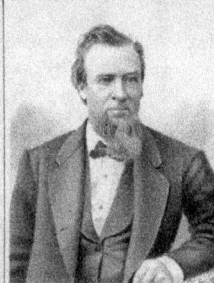

Hon. J. C. BURBANK.
St. Paul.

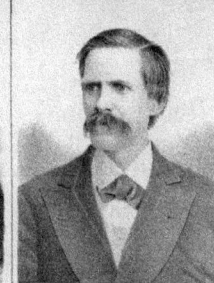

Hon. W. P. MURRAY.
St. Paul.

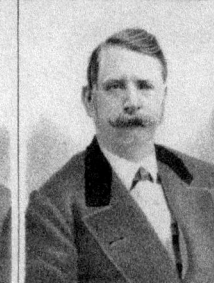

Hon. GEO. L. BECKER.
St. Paul.

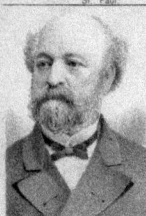

A. H. CATHCART.
St. Paul.

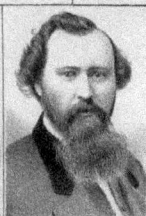

J. W. CATHCART.
St. Paul.

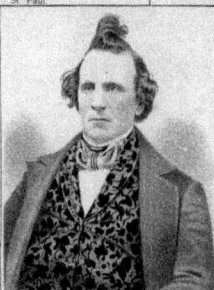

Hon. LYMAN DAYTON.
St. Paul.

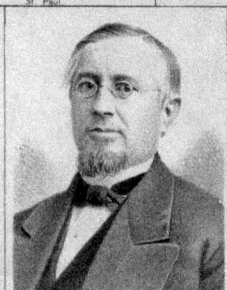

Hon. HENRY L. MOSS.
St. Paul.

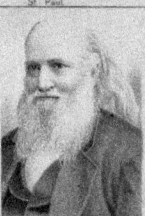

A. T. C. PIERSON.
St. Paul.

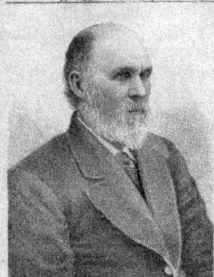

J. R. IRVIN.
St. Paul.

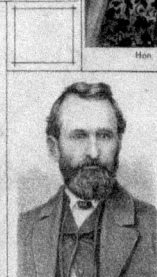

GEO. G. STEVENS.
Rushford.

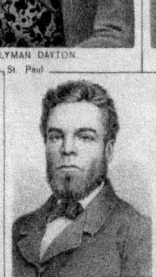

Hon. C. F. BUCK.
Winona.

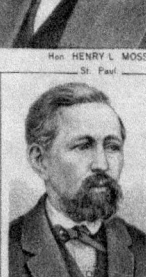

S. S. STEBBINS.
Rushford.

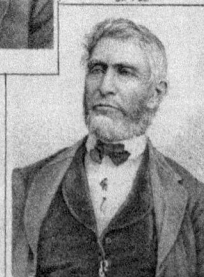

ANSON NORTHUP.
Duluth.

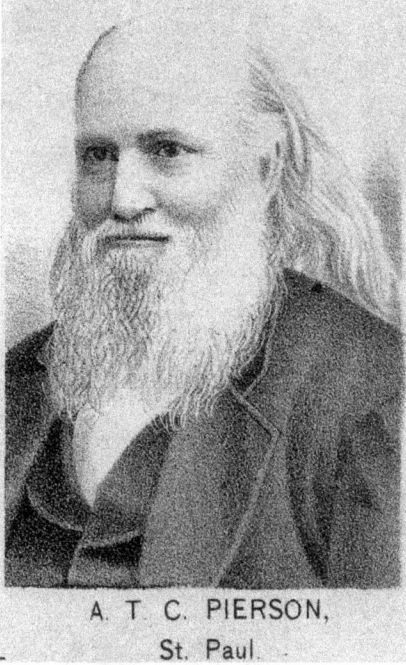

A. T. C. PIERSON,
St. Paul.

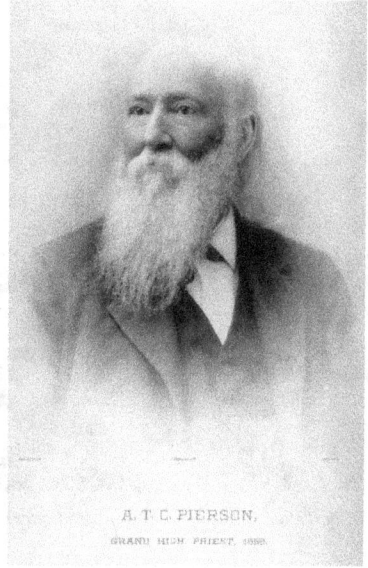

A. T. C. PIERSON,
GRAND HIGH PRIEST, 1885.

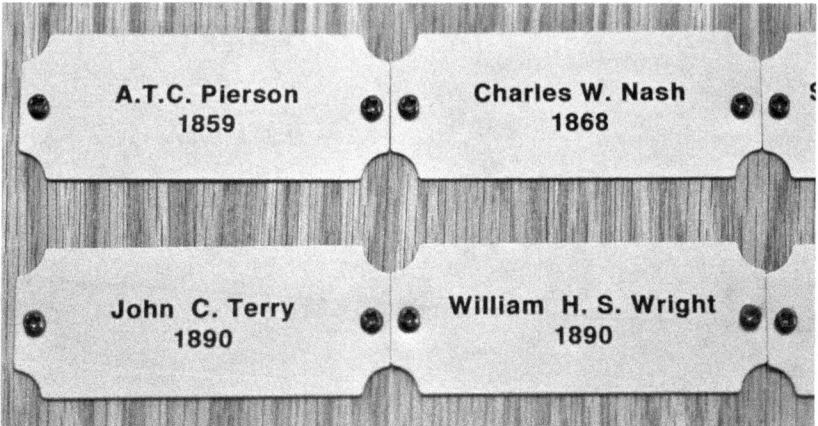

| A.T.C. Pierson 1859 | Charles W. Nash 1868 | |
| John C. Terry 1890 | William H. S. Wright 1890 | |

47

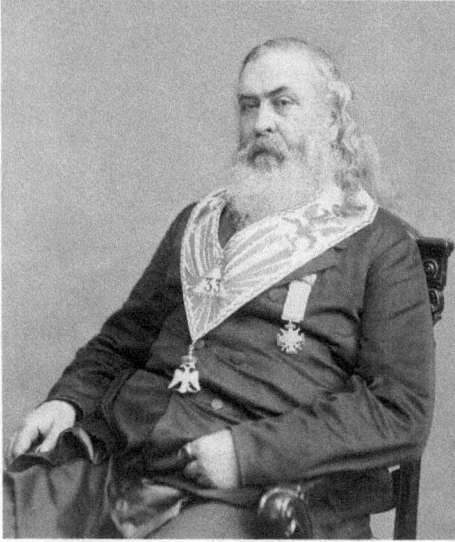

Albert Pike, Sovereign Grand Commander.

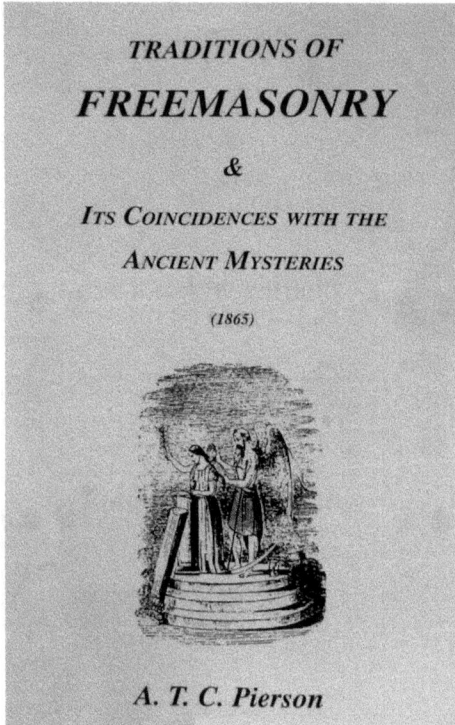

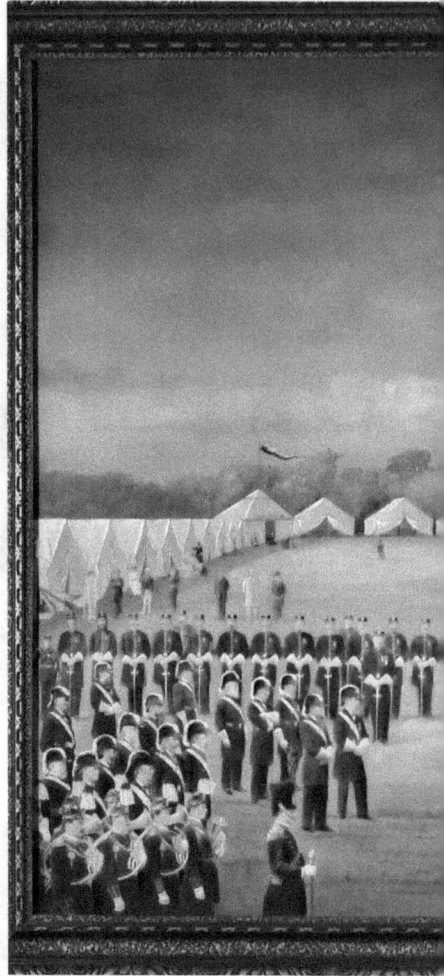

TRADITIONS OF

FREEMASONRY

&

ITS COINCIDENCES WITH THE
ANCIENT MYSTERIES

(1865)

A. T. C. Pierson

Hand-colored photograph of Damascus Commandry at White Bear Lake by artist and photographer Charles A. Zimmerman.

Pierson's first book.

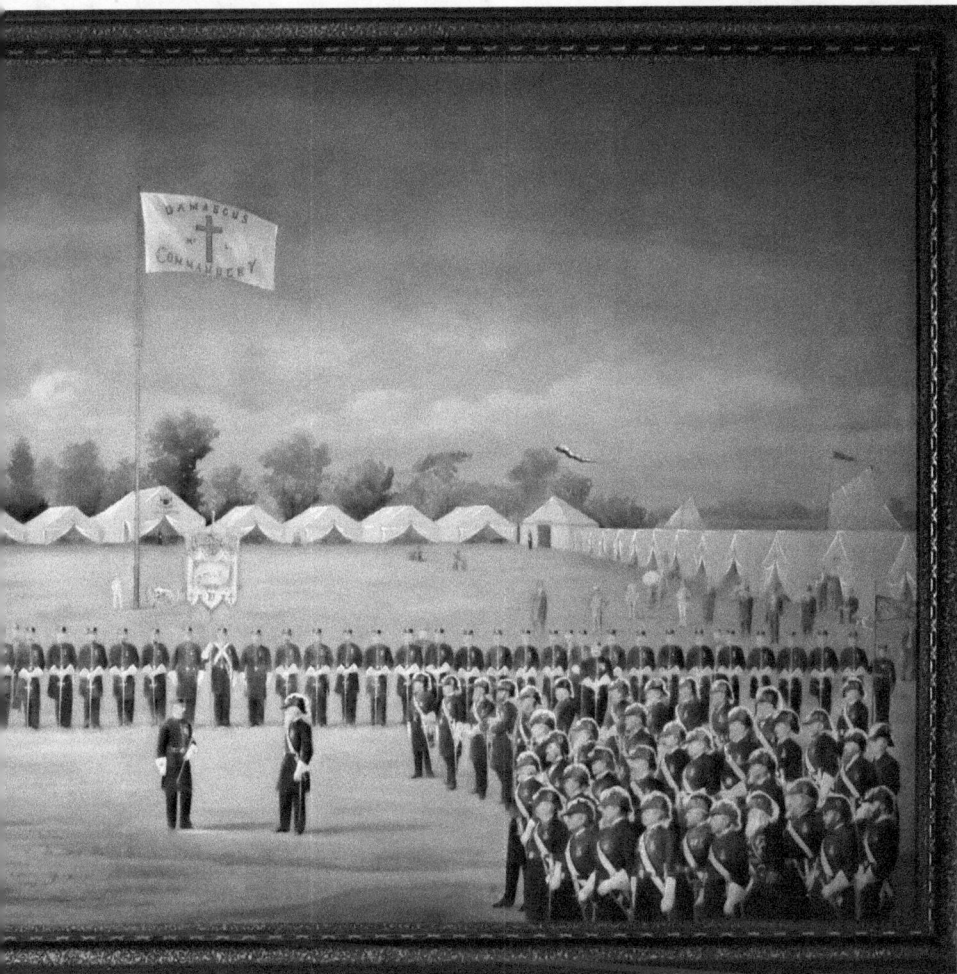

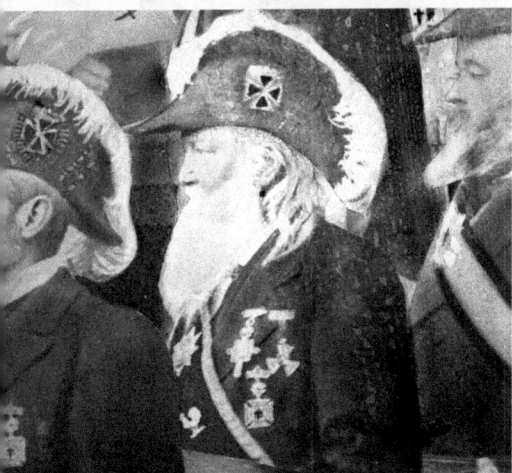

Close-up shows Pierson near bottom right corner.

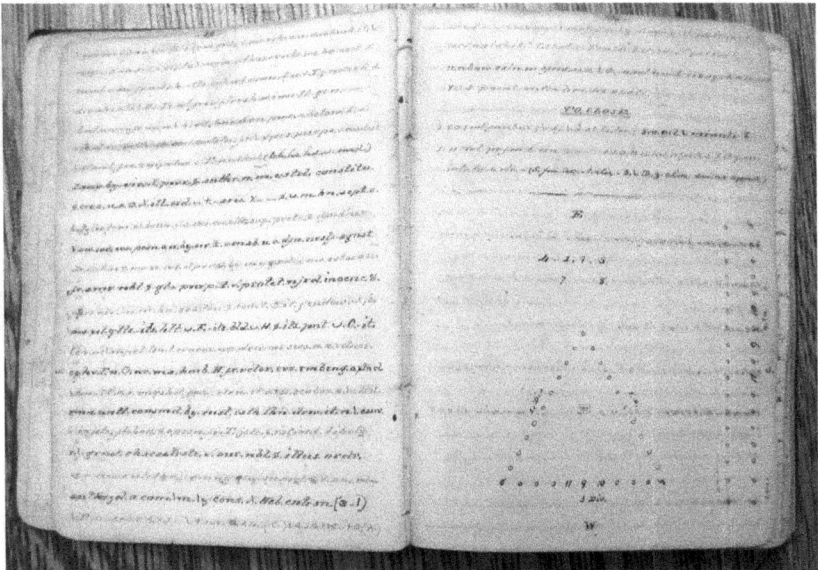

Handwritten ritual by A.T.C. Pierson.

Handwritten cipher by A.T.C. Pierson.

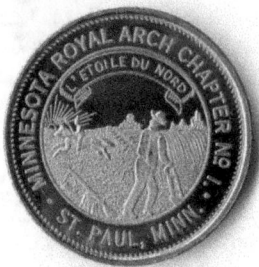

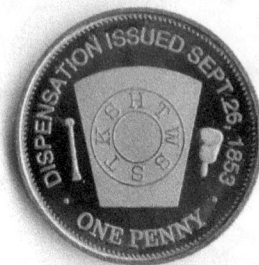

Minnesota Chapter #1 RAM Chapter Penny showing Minnesota state seal.

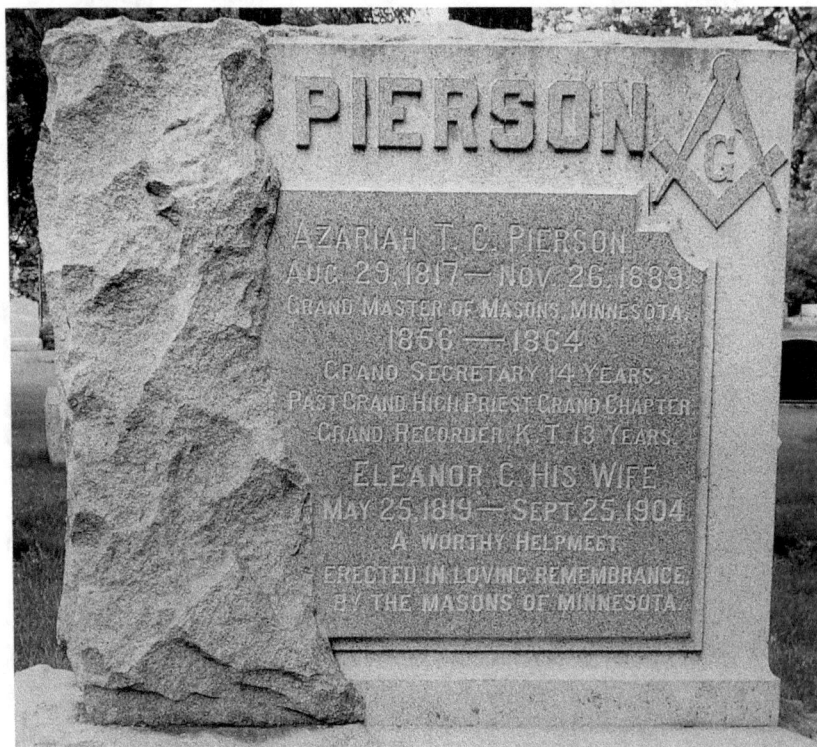

The rough and smooth ashlar monument on A.T.C. and Eleanor Pierson's grave at Oakland Cemetery in Saint Paul, Minnesota.

Appendix 1

A Brief Sketch of the Beginnings of Minnesota Chapter Number 1, RAM

By Charles W. Nelson P.H.P.
Sept. 7, 2003

The first meeting of Royal Arch Masons in the Territory of Minnesota was convened in the office of General George L. Becker, later first president of the St. Paul and Pacific Railroad, 198 West Third Street, in Saint Paul during the month of July 1853. There were eight men present and their purpose was to organize a chapter of Royal Arch Masons in St. Paul. The group comprised prominent early settlers and community leaders: Azariah Theodore Crane Pierson, Henry Morris, Henry Buel, J.J. Bardwell, William H. Newton, George W. Biddle, and Charles D, Fillmore.

Application for dispensation was made to the General Grand Chapter of the United States under the name of Minnesota Royal Arch Chapter No. 1. In order to proceed with the application, favorable recommendation from a duly chartered Chapter was required. Accordingly, Comp. Pierson journeyed to Dubuque, Iowa, to gain support, and being successful, he forwarded the application to M.E. Willis Stewart, soon to be elected Deputy General Grand High Priest. At the Triennial Convocation, the General Grand Chapter granted Minnesota's request and issued dispensation on Sept. 26, 1853. The first officers designated by Stewart were A.T.C. Pierson as High Priest, Judge Andrew G. Chatfield as King, and George L. Becker as Scribe.

Work in the new Chapter commenced on Dec. 21, 1853. The Chapter opened on the Royal Arch Degree for the purpose of electing four additional Companions to make a total of sixteen founding members under dispensation. These founders, with their respective occupations and places of residence were:

Azariah Theodore Crane Pierson, Indian agent, St. Paul
Andrew G. Chatfield, U.S. District judge, Belle Plaine
George L. Becker, lawyer, St. Paul
Henry Morris, accountant, St. Paul
Andrew J. Whitney, accountant, St. Paul
George W. Biddle, dentist, St. Paul
Norris Hobart, clergyman, Ramsey County
William H. Newton, real estate dealer, St. Paul
Charles D. Fillmore, carpenter, St. Paul
Sylvanus Patridge, merchant, Stillwater
Daniel Mc Lane, lumberman, Stillwater
Abram Van Vohres, surveyor, Stillwater
Alfred E. Ames, physician, Minneapolis
Emmanuel Case, farmer, Minneapolis
Henry Buel, merchant, St. Paul
Andrew J. Morgan, painter. St. Paul

Thirty Companions were exalted during the period of dispensation, making a total membership of 64 at the time of Charter.

The Chapter adopted a portion of the Constitution of the Grand Chapter of Michigan as a guide for its organization and protocol. Nearly three years later, application was made for a Charter, which was promptly granted on September 11, 1856, by the General Grand Chapter, meeting in Hartford, Connecticut.

The first meeting of Minnesota Royal Arch Chapter No. 1 under Charter was held on Wednesday evening, November 12, 1856, with Companion Reverend John Penman (exalted April 15, 1856) presiding. Election was held and ballots cast, resulting in the installation of Comp. Pierson as High Priest, an office that he held until June 1859.

During his tenure, 68 Companions had been exalted and 16 joining from other chapter jurisdictions.

The industry and zeal of the early companions of the Minnesota Chapter is remarkable to the chronicler of its history. On the first meeting of the chapter under dispensation, December 21, 1853, three candidates — D.W. Dunwell, a carpenter, James Y. Caldwell, also a carpenter, and Peter T. Bradley, a harness-maker, all from St. Paul — were presented for admission, advanced to the Degree of Mark Master, and summarily inducted into the Oriental Chair. One week later these aspirants were received and acknowledged as Most Excellent Masters and exalted as Royal Arch Masons. One petitioner, by virtue of having presided as Master of his Lodge, was inducted as a Past Master without the obligatory degree. In yet another instance, Comp. William Freeborn, a land agent from Red Wing, presented his petition on February 15th of 1854 and received all of the degrees the same evening because he was about to return to his home, a day's travel distant.

The Chapter in these first years met in a rented hall on the third floor of the building where it had initially met in George Becker's office to request dispensation. It was then sharing quarters with Saint Paul Lodge No. 3, and on February 22, 1854, accepted Ancient Landmark Lodge No. 5 as another tenant. On April 5, 1854, a committee was appointed to meet with various lodges (Masonic and otherwise) to explore the possibility of erecting a building for all to meet. In May of that year, Excellent. Comp. Pierson went east to receive the Order of High Priesthood. During his absence, a special convocation was called to receive two visitors, Past High Priests from Maine and Iowa.

Although the Chapter met somewhat irregularly during its infancy, Pierson kept meticulous records. He officiated at virtually every installation of officers and was instrumental in drafting the regulations for the governance of the Chapter. It may be of interest that the prescribed date of the annual meeting of the Chapter was to be the stated meeting immediately preceding the Festival of St. John the Baptist. Two standing committees were formed: Finance and Accounts and Charity in Relief. As to eligibility for membership:

> "No candidate can be exalted unless he has been a Master Mason at least three months, and made suitable proficiency, and resided within the jurisdiction of this Chapter (which at present includes the whole territory of Minnesota) six months, provided however this section as to residence is not to apply to Master Masons, members of subordinate Lodges within the Territory and who so resided at the formation of this Chapter."

The annual dues were fixed at two dollars, with the fees for degrees set at five dollars Mark master, five dollars past master, five dollars most excellent master and $10 Royal arch. The regulations mandated that "only 2° can be conferred on any one candidate at the same meeting, unless an extraordinary case, but which shall be decided by a photo of the chapter."

In the early years, there was some irregularity in election of officers. The first election under Charter took place on Nov. 12, 1856, however no other election took place until June 2, 1858. As such, Pierson served his first term as High Priest for one year and seven months. It was also often the case that the veilsmen were not installed, or the actual installation was neglected, with officers simply proclaimed in their positions.

The finances were primarily for rent and the purchase of furnishings and paraphernalia, at first of a makeshift variety. On Feb. 10, 1858, the offices of Treasurer and Secretary were confirmed with the election of Comp. Norman W, Kittson, who listed his occupation as Indian Trader, as Treasurer and W. S. Combs as Secretary. The Chapter assumed the responsibility of fitting up the quarters, including all furniture, heat and lights and to apportion the costs to the others sharing the hall. Other expenses included a bill for $44.40, which covered rent, sawing and carrying wood, drayage for moving Chapter furniture, purchase of wood, fixing up the tabernacle, and fitting up the room. The Chapter's portion of the rent for the hall amounted to $135 a year. Kittson initiated a program to estimate the total yearly expenses and to apportion them among the tenants accordingly. This was the beginning of the Chapter budget and a means of simplifying accounting.

On Sept. 7, 1859, Minnesota Chapter was honored to receive Albert G. Mackey, M.D., Grand High Priest of the Grand Royal Arch Chapter of South Carolina. On this occasion, Mackey conferred the Royal Arch Degree. A noted author and scholar, Mackey was considered the highest authority on Masonry in the county.

During the Civil War, the Chapter continued to meet but was well aware of the patriotic obligations of its members. A dispensation from the Grand Chapter, signed by Alfred E. Ames, Grand High Priest, and received on March 27, 1862, empowered Minnesota Chapter to receive the petitions, act upon the same, and confer the degrees at discretion upon Brothers L. L. Baxter, a lawyer, and Charles Johnson, a farmer, both from Carver. These men belonged to the Regular Army and were under marching orders to leave the state in a few days. They were exalted on April 11, 1862. Also, the Chapter conducted funeral services on Companion Captain William Henry Acker (exalted March 25, 1857) who fell in the Battle of Pittsburg Landing. The Companions of St. Anthony Chapter No. 3 also attended. Frequently, the Chapter room was draped in mourning during this period. Because of the Civil War, the meeting of the General Grand Chapter in Memphis, Tennessee, in 1862 was canceled.

On April 21, 1868, at 3:00 a.m., the Mackubin Building, which had been occupied by the Chapter and several other Masonic bodies, burned, and the Charter and other properties of the Chapter were lost. Offers of assistance were made by the St. Paul Lodge No. 2 of the Odd Fellows, St. John's Chapter No. 7, Minneapolis, and St. Anthony Falls Chapter No. 3. The May 7, 1868, Chapter meeting was held at the Odd Fellows Hall, and the next year entered into a lease for quarters in the Forepaugh Block at the corner of Wabasha and Third Streets.

In outfitting the new hall, the Chapter purchased a total of $665.63 of paraphernalia. It is of interest to sample a few of these items and costs. A set of costumes cost $350.00; a set of twelve officers jewels, $48.00; a signet ring, $4.00; a set of five swords and belts, $62.50; a brass incense burner, $15.00; a pot of manna and Aaron's rod, $5.25; an Ark of the Covenant, $20.00, and a set of officers aprons $60.00.

On June 3, 1869, the annual convocation was held and a new corps of officers elected and installed. A new book was purchased for the records of the Chapter, the previous minute's book being opened on Nov. 12, 1856, and used for 13 years. The Chapter would continue to keep a minute record of its proceedings, finances, rosters of officers, and work in an archival treasure spanning 150 years. This brief sketch has been intended to bring to light but a few of the stories concealed therein. Taken in context, the history of Minnesota Chapter No. 1 is the history of Masonry in Minnesota.

In 1903, looking back over the early years of the Chapter and the lives of those who are among its founders, Excellent Companion William S. Combs, a St. Paul bookseller exalted on Jan. 3, 1855, made the following observation in the florid prose of the era:

> "This is an age of history making and history recording, and consequently an age of rapid progress along all lines of human endeavor. The historic ages as compared with the prehistoric age of this planet is but a span, but the rate of progress into civilization of the races of the Earth in this age is marvelous, and can be accounted for in no other."

Appendix 2

The following an excerpt from a paper read by William S. Combs of St. Paul at the banquet following the annual assembly of the Grand Council, Royal and Select Master, held in Minneapolis on Oct. 12, 1903, with some added information furnished by the grand recorder.

"The American Tyler" Dec. 15, 1903

Cryptic Masonry in Minnesota

Some time during the year 1868, Compo A.T.C. Pierson, while on a visit to New York, secured a dispensation from the Grand Council of Royal and Select Masters of New York, or from the Grand Master thereof, to communicate the degrees of the Cryptic Rite upon such Royal Arch Masons in Minnesota as he might choose, with a view of forming a council. He selected for the honors the following companions of St. Paul, and possibly others: John C. Terry, Samuel Willey, Isaac P. Wright, Chas. W. Nash, Geo. W. Prescott, George L. Otis, Wm. S. Combs, Josiah Marvin and C. W. Carpenter. After he had communicated the degrees to the above named companions, a council was formed and officers chosen. Compo John C. Terry was installed as Thrice Illustrious Master and Compo Wm. S. Combs, recorder. The council procured from Compo Geo. W. Seymour of Taylor's Falls a copy of the New York ritual, and in due time, conferred the degrees upon a number of companions under authority of the aforesaid dispensation. When the time came to apply for a charter, Companion Pierson refused to meet with or assist us, claiming that the Ancient and Accepted Scottish Rite for the Southern Jurisdiction, of which he was then an officer, had jurisdiction over the degrees of Royal and Select Master, and that consequently he was debarred from taking any further interest in our council. As a matter of fact, Companion Pierson, as such officer, communicated the degrees to several other Royal Arch Masons in St. Paul, who were subsequently healed and admitted into St. Paul Council. Being thus deprived of the assistance of Companion Pierson, I was urgently requested by the other companions of our Council to apply to the Grand Council of Iowa for a charter.

Appendix 3

In reply to a remark of Comp. Melish of Ohio, Editor of the Masonic Review, to the effect that the Council Degrees of the Scottish Rite have no affinity whatever with those of the York Rite. A.C.T. Pierson said:

"'Never too old to learn.' Here we find the proclamation of a new set of Council Degrees; new of course, if those practiced in Ohio have no affinity with the Council Degrees of the Scottish Rite!

"York Rite Council Degrees! We have always supposed that the York Rite was confined to three degrees.

"Among the manuscripts brought to this country by the refugees from St. Domingo were rituals of the Select and Royal Master; side degrees given by Inspector Generals of the 33° A. and A. Rite, by virtue of their rank. After the formation of the Supreme Council at Charleston, Myers deposited with it various rituals; among them was the only known copy of the Select and Royal Degrees.

"Philip Eckel, of Baltimore, was a member of the Supreme Council.

"In the peregrinations of Jeremy L. Cross on his lecturing tours, he went to Baltimore. Eckel communicated the degrees to Cross, with authority to communicate them to Royal Arch Masons. On his return north, Cross communicated the degrees, charging five dollars for them — the older Masons in Maryland believe that Cross was expelled for so doing — and established

Councils in New York, Connecticut, &c. All the Councils in the Northern States, to-day, and several of those in the Southern, can trace their 'genealogy' back to Council No. 1, in Connecticut, established by Jeremy L. Cross.

"The Supreme Council of the northern jurisdiction never claimed or exercised any authority over the degrees, and a few years since the Southern Supreme Council formally relinquished its rights. The A. and A. system is perfect in itself; it requires no side degrees to explain any of its degrees, and as the Select and Royal Degrees did not, and could not, throw any light, and having no use for them, but rather a source for vexation and bother, the Southern Supreme Council just incontinently threw them aside, to be picked up by any that chose.

"We will add, that the degrees, when properly given, are pretty and elucidative, and being so intimately connected with the Royal Arch, should be given by the Chapter after the M.E. degree."

Appendix 4

A.T.C. Pierson's Funeral Preparations, Service, and Eulogy

Brethren of the Grand Lodge, I have called you together today in special communication, for the purpose of performing a most solemn duty.

Bro. A. T. C. Pierson, P∴ G∴ M∴ of this jurisdiction and for the past fourteen years R∴ W∴ Grand Secretary of this Grand Lodge, departed this life at 3 o'clock in the morning of the 26th, in the seventy-third year of his age.

We meet today to consign his remains to their last resting place on Earth, agreeably to the ancient forms and ceremonies of our fraternity. Bro. Pierson has held worthily the highest official honors that Masonry can confer.

He was the most learned, most honored and most widely known Mason in the Northwest. In every department, field, and branch of Masonry, he was a most skilled and master workman. He had devoted his life to the good cause of Masonry, and died at his post with his pen almost literally in his hand. His patriarchal presence, his genial smile, his fraternal greetings, his sage counsels, we shall enjoy no more on Earth forever.

For what he did in life for Masonry, especially in this jurisdiction, let there be lasting and grateful remembrance. At some future time, we shall pay a fuller and more fitting tribute to his memory.

Solemn labors now claim our immediate attention. As soon as informed of the demise of Bro. Pierson, the necessary steps were taken to provide for his proper and fitting burial. A meeting of the presiding officers of the different local lodges of this city was held yesterday with I. B. B. Sprague, Master of Ancient Landmark Lodge, as chairman, and local committees were appointed. The General Supervisory Committee consists of:

Bro. I. B. B. Sprague, Ancient Landmark Lodge, Chairman; Dr. George R. Metcalf, K. P. Cullen, St. Paul Lodge; George Brookings, Braden Lodge; John Dale, Shekinah Lodge; Walter Holcomb, Summit Lodge; W. M. Todd, Midway Lodge; W. P. Jewett, High Priest of Minnesota Royal Arch Chapter; E.C. Merrill, High Priest of Summit Royal Arch Chapter;

W.H. Sanborn, Grand Commander of Knights Templar; W. M. Bushnell, Eminent Commander of Damascus Commandery, No. 1; W. H. S. Wright, Eminent Commander of Paladin, No. 21; Sir Knights R. C. Munger and George S. Acker.

The Grand Commandery Knights Templar and subordinate commanderies will act as escort to the Grand Lodge.

The Grand Chapter Royal Arch Masons will also assist in the ceremonies and join in the procession. The procession will be formed by Bro. George S. Acker, Acting Grand Marshal, and proceed to the residence of our deceased brother, and bear from thence his remains to the Peoples Church, where religious services will be conducted by Bro. S. G. Smith, our Grand Orator, and thence we shall proceed to Oakland Cemetery, and with the honors of Masonry, consign the remains of our venerable brother to their Mother Earth.

I have designated as pall bearers, P∴ G∴ Masters H. R. Wells, Chas. Griswold, C. H. Benton, H. R. Denny, E. W. Durant, P∴ S∴ G∴ W∴ S. E. Adams, and Past Masters W. P. Murray and Freeman James.

The services at the grave were conducted by the M∴ W∴ Grand Master and the purposes of the special communication having been completed the Grand Lodge returned to Masonic Hall and was duly closed at 5:30 P.M.

J. A. Kiester, Grand Master.

Attest: Thomas Montgomery, Grand Secretary.

"But we meet today, brethren, surrounded by the somber habili-
ments of mourning. What means this? Alas! One of our number is
missing. The fraternal chain is broken. A venerable presence, always
recognized here at this hour in our annual assemblies during thirty-
six years past, appears not among us today. A light has gone out!
Father Pierson, for so many years our R.'. W.'. Grand Secretary, is
no more with us. His earthly labors done, he has gone forward and
entered upon the next stage of the sublime travel of immortality. At
three o'clock in the morning of the twenty-sixth day of November
last, he quietly and in peace departed this life. The morning of that
day broke, for him, on the other shore—the dawn, we can confidently
hope, of a brighter day than this Earth can ever know.

No, he is not with us today, but has gone to attend that vast
assembly of the people of all ages, nations, kindreds and tongues,
gathered and gathering in that mysterious land which lies beyond
the bounds of this mortal life, and from whose bourne no traveler
ever returns. And 'There's a mansion and a welcome and a multitude
is there, Who have met upon the Level, and been tried upon the
Square.'

Among all the dead of those who have held official position in this
Grand Lodge, and among all the deceased of the craft in this jurisdiction, his demise is the one of largest significance, in a masonic sense.

His name has been a familiar one throughout the American
masonic world for many years, and he has been connected in a
prominent way with all the masonic organizations of this state from
their beginning. Yet he was not only thus known; but in the families
of many of the brethren in our large jurisdiction, even the children
were familiar with and kindly spake the name of "Grandfather
Pierson."

He was a member of the first masonic lodge organized in this city, which was named St. Paul Lodge. In 1854, he assisted in the organization of Ancient Landmark Lodge, No. 5, of this city, and was a charter member thereof.

He had also prepared an elaborate work on masonic jurisprudence, the manuscript of which, unhappily, was destroyed by fire before the publication of the book, and he had not, as he once told me, the heart to write it over.

As a Mason of long experience, of official services in every branch of Masonry, and of wide and varied learning, Bro. Pierson had few equals and no superiors.

He accompanied us during the summer at the laying of the corner stones at Sauk Centre, Litchfield and Duluth, and expressed himself as greatly enjoying these excursions. He also, in October last, attended the Triennial Grand Encampment of Knights Templar at Washington, D. C.

He was buried on the twenty-ninth day of November last in Oakland Cemetery, near this city. I deem it unnecessary here to enter into all the detail of the funeral. It is sufficient to say that he was interred according to our solemn ceremonies, under the auspices of this Grand Lodge; the Grand Commandery of Knights Templar and many subordinate commanderies, under command of R∴ E∴ Sir W. H. Sanborn, Grand Commander, acting as escort to the Grand Lodge; the Grand Chapter of Royal Arch Masons of the state, and many lodges, and hundreds of Masons, and many citizens, joining in the largest and most splendid funeral procession ever known in the state — a grand and most impressive tribute of respect to the memory of our deceased brother. And as the sun of that day was setting and the shades of evening rapidly gathering, we laid him to his final rest. His life on Earth was done, the day was done, and our solemn labors also done.

Bro. Pierson is survived by his venerable wife and three daughters, one unmarried, one the widow of the late Major Hatch, and one the

widow of the late James V. Caldwell, besides a number of grandchil-
dren and great-grandchildren. It is hardly necessary, brethren, in a
lodge of Masons, to say it, but the widow and the fatherless are in our
special care and remembrance."

-J. A. Kiester, Grand Master.

Select Bibliography:

Traditions of Freemasonry and its Coincidences with the Ancient Mysteries by A.T.C. Pierson

History of the Supreme Council 33 1861-1891 by James Carter, 33

Chief Hole-In-The-Day and the 1862 Chippewa Disturbance, a reappraisal by Mark Diedrich

Masonic Sketch Book and Gleanings from the Harvest Field of Masonic Literature by Edwin Du Laurans.

History of Ramsey County and the City of St. Paul by George E. Warner and Charles M. Foote

The Scottish Rite of Freemasonry in Minnesota 1867-2001

Pen Pictures of St. Paul and Biographical Sketches of Old Settlers 1859 by T.M. Newson

History of St. Paul and Vicinity by Henry Anson Castle

Lights and Shadows of St. Paul Lodge No. 3, A. F. & A. M., 1849-1949

Annual Report of the Commissioner of Indian Affairs

The American Tyler-Keystone

Various Proceedings from Grand Lodges and Grand Chapters

American Photographs: The First Century by Merry A. Foresta

Author Bio

Ray Hayward began his health maintenance and Martial Arts training in 1973, studying Kenpo Karate and Jiu-Jitsu. In 1977, Ray met and began to study with Master T.T. Liang in Boston and learned the complete Yang Style T'ai-Chi Ch'uan system, as well as Praying Mantis, Ch'i-Kung, Taoist Meditation, Ch'in-Na, Wu Dang Sword and various weapons. In 1984, Ray moved to Minnesota to continue studying with Master Liang, where he passed through a formal ceremony to become an inner-door disciple of Master T.T. Liang. Ray is a published author and has written articles and several books about Master Liang's life and teachings.

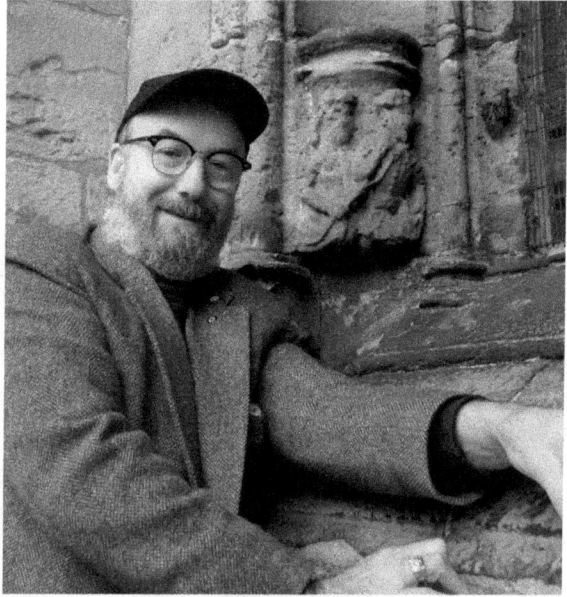

Since 1994, Ray has been a student under Grandmaster Wai-lun Choi, the lineage holder of the Luk Hop Bat Fat kung-fu style. He continues to study and sponsor workshops at his academy with Master Choi and has written several articles and a book titled *Real Gold Does Not Fear The Fire, the teachings of Grandmaster Wai-lun Choi.*

For more than 40 years, Ray has studied Taoist Meditation, Alchemy, and Sexual Yoga with such masters as Paul Gallagher, Kenneth Cohen, and many others. He currently studies the breath techniques and cold-exposure training of Wim Hof and Stig Severinson, and Modern Tactical Martial Arts with Master Rob Jones.

In London in 1989, Ray took Bayat, an initiation into the Naqshbandi Sufi Order, with the 40th Grandshaykh, Moulana Shaykh Nazim Al-Haqqani. He directed a Sufi meditation center in Minneapolis for more than seven years under Shaykh Nazim's guidance and authority.

Ray has also studied Hypnotherapy and Psychology with Lourae Becker, and is certified in the Healing Tao System by Loretta Robb. He has made extensive research and study concerning the Western Mysteries, including Alchemy, Freemasonry, the Knights Templar, the Rosicrucians, Druidry, Celtic history, and Rosslyn Chapel. Ray studied in Scotland as an apprentice under WB Joe Lang, the foremost authority on Rosslyn Chapel and was authorized by him to give the teachings and tours of the Chapel and surrounding sacred sites.

For many years, Ray has had the honor of being a student of Judge David Sinclair Bouschor, the founder of Clan Sinclair USA, a Past Grandmaster of Freemasonry, and a Knight Templar.

Ray has been knighted into several Knight Templar Orders including;

Masonic Knights Templar, knighted by Grand Commander Charles W. Nelson

Knight Templar Order of Light and Wisdom, knighted by Brother Amaldreth

O.S.T.I. Order of Sovereign Templar Initiates, knighted by Grandmaster Timothy W. Hogan

Cathar Knights of the Ordre Chevalier Faydits Colombe du Paraclete, knighted by Grandmaster Tau Sendagovious

O.T.I. Knights Templar, knighted by Chevalier Paul Sanda

Masonic Offices held include:

Past Master of Braden Lodge 168, 2006

Past High Priest of Minnesota Chapter No. 1, Royal Arch Masons, 2004 and 2005

Past Commander of Damascus Commandery No. 1, Knights Templar, 2005 and 2006

Right Eminent Past Grand Commander of the Grand Commandery of Knights Templar of Minnesota, 2011-2012

V.E. Preceptor of Good Samaritan Tabernacle, Holy Royal Arch Knights Templar Priests 2018

In 2010, Ray became a Druid Graduate in the Order of Bards, Ovates, and Druids. He has traveled to Pennsylvania, Upstate N.Y. and Glastonbury, U.K. to study directly with the Chosen Chief of the Order, Philip Carr-Gomm. He currently guides a Seed-group of Druids in the Twin Cities area.

Ray Hayward is dedicated to the spiritual journey known as the "Grail Quest." He sees the need for personal understanding, and self-awareness to be able to affect the conditions and changes needed for world peace. He feels that to be awake, empowered, and self-realized are the keys to a harmonious life.

Contacts

Ray Hayward's Blog: The Inspired Teacher
http://www.rayhayward.com/

Ray Hayward's Books
http://www.lulu.com/spotlight/Ray_Hayward

Grand Lodge of Minnesota
https://mn-masons.org/

Grand Chapter of Minnesota
http://www.mnyorkrite.org/grand-chapter.html

Grand Commandery of Minnesota
http://www.mnyorkrite.org/grand-commandery.html

Timothy Hogan
http://www.lulu.com/spotlight/Emerys

Minnesota Historical Society
http://www.mnhs.org/

Julie Cisler (graphic design & production)
juliecisler13@hotmail.com